# Crockpot Recipes

## Scrumptious Crock Pot and Slow Cooker Recipes

Janet Daley

# Table of Contents

# Introduction

Enter the new era of slow cooking and find the answers to healthy, convenient and flavor-rich foods. Steeped in their own juices and contained in a temperature regulated environment, contents are allowed to keep many of their vitamins, normally lost through boiling and baking methods. As society wakes up and sees the negative effects that greasy and fast foods have on the human body, crock pots are making a huge comeback. If you are one of the thousands that are looking to improve your health, keep meals simple, and enjoy the succulent flavor of foods, this book is just for you.

Learn how almost any type of meal can be created by using your crock pot. Not limited to meats and stews, you will discover how fruits and vegetables can retain a rich and fascinating flavor. Green beans, carrots and peppers will keep their natural juices and nutrients, then wrap their wonderful flavor around other added foods. By using spices and herbs, see how new and exciting creations can rejuvenate classic dishes.

Create new foods from scratch, like yogurt and applesauce, or make movie night a special occasion with cinnamon almonds, that are warm and atomic. Learn how to prepare fresh vegetables, or entire meals, for storage, once the growing season is over. There are also many treats that are shown in this book that you never dreamed could be made with a slow cooker. The rich flavors that are held within your crock pot, and slow cooked to perfection, will convince you that crock pots are here to stay.

When crock pots were first introduced in the early 1970s, their purpose was one of time saving meal preparation. By placing a chicken or roast in the slow cooker in the morning, you could find a tender, tasty main meal, hours later. Unfortunately, the crock pot was forced to compete with the emerging microwave oven and drive-through restaurants. What seemed an easier and more grandiose way of eating, the crock pot was quietly stored on a shelf. It is time to pull out that amazing piece of cookware and learn how to make your life easier, healthier and create better tasting meals.

To get back into the swing of things, a 5-day meal planner has been included, along with tips for purchasing a crockpot. While your old model may work just fine, discover the updates and additional features that have been added over the past 40 years. Read about the benefits of slow cooking and how those with little practice in cooking, can create gourmet foods. While the microwave is still a handy tool in everyday living, you will find that your crock pot has an important place on your kitchen counter.

# Chapter 1: Benefits of Crockpot Cooking

Back in 1100 A.D., slow cooking consisted of digging a hole in the earth and warming the pit with wood and coal.  As society graduated to wood-burning stoves, then ovens, this procedure is still known to keep foods rich in taste.  The crockpot is the ultimate way to benefit from this long-standing tradition of healthy eating and enjoying flavorful meals.

Crockpot cooking allows you to place tough cuts of beef in a controlled, temperature-regulated environment, where the sides and bottom emit heat and baste the contents in their own juices.  The past forty years have introduced different foods, like vegetables, fruits and grains that also reveal a succulent flavor by using this method.

Creative minds have further come up with ways to prepare entire meals in advance, freeze, and 'throw in the pot', returning in hours to a ready-made dinner that is convenient and healthy.  Fresh foods are always the best way to eat, but the convenience of canned and boxed foodstuffs have drawn a fast-paced society away from eating right.  The crock pot is a great way to get back into nutritional eating, plus save time.

Most crock pots have a separate lining that makes

cleanup simple. By removing the ceramic pot, washing is a snap. Many models are also dishwasher safe. Using several pots and pans for cooking can put a damper on any thought of meal preparation. A crock pot eliminates the needless worry of the daunting task of after-meal cleanup.

The simplicity of a crock pot keeps maintenance to a minimum. Crockpots are moderately priced and come with an operators manual and where to find replacement parts. The extravagance of electronics today, can break a budget in repairing cooking appliances. The crock pot offers a simple alternative.

Energy-efficiency is on everyone's mind, and the crock pot serves as a wonderful way to cut back on energy consumption.
Having a crock pot turned on for 8 hours, uses approximately 0.8 kWh. Using an oven for 1 ½ hrs, to prepare the same dish, uses around 3.0 kWh. The crockpot is one of the greenest appliances you can own.

Different sizes and features make slow cookers family friendly. From 3-quart to 7-quart, and larger, you can determine the number of people you wish to feed. Some models are programmable for extended cooking or shutting off at a specified time. The temperature varies little with models, ranging from 170 degrees F to 280 degrees F.

Tender meats, succulent flavors, ease of preparation,

energy-efficient, and an assortment of models makes slow cooking sensible, besides beneficial.

# Chapter 2: Tips and Information for Slow Cooking

Here are 10 tips for making your crock pot cooking even easier. By knowing how certain foods react to slow cooking can prepare you on making the perfect dishes.

Never overfill. Crockpots are designed to heat halfway up the sides for even cooking. For this reason, filling a pot more than ½ full, can have an adverse effect on the overall quality.

Do not add water to a recipe unless specifically asked for. Many foods contain natural juices that will seep during cooking. By adding more liquid, you may dilute the taste.

When possible, wait until the last 30 minutes of crockpot cooking before adding milk products. Dairy products can break down and actually increase the cooking temperature inside the pot.

Frozen meats can be placed directly in the crockpot for cooking. However, always add 1 cup of warm liquid to the pot before adding the frozen meat. Also add an additional 2 hours high temperature cooking to these foods.

Long-grained rice or risotto give the best results for

grains prepared in a crockpot. Also, taking a little longer to slow cook, add water as needed.

The 'high' setting on a crockpot does not mean that a higher heat is reached, just that it takes a shorter amount of time to reach an approximate 210 degree F simmer point. When cooking on 'high' cut the recommended time in half. For instances, if a recipe calls for cooking 8 hours, check for doneness in 4 hours.

Never preheat your crock pot.

Shellfish will overcook easily. It is recommended to add shellfish to a crockpot 15 to 20 minutes before serving to keep it firm and not overdone.

Any type of pasta should be boiled on the stove top. Place in the slow cooker with the rest of the ingredients, 30 minutes before completion.

When using herbs and spices, use half the amount at the beginning of the cooking cycle, and add the rest toward the end. This will help keep the flavors more intense.

Read your instruction manual carefully. Many glass lids are not dishwasher-safe, although the ceramic container may be.

The crock pot is a wonderful way to prepare fresh foods for storage. Making applesauce, preparing pumpkin puree, and making your own yogurt are a few ways that slow cooking can stretch those fresh foods.  Fresh pumpkin is plentiful  in the fall, and a great way to store up for the winter.  Follow these tips on preparing and freezing pumpkin, and you will always have plenty of fresh pumpkin puree on hand.

While you may think that large pumpkins have the best meat for pies, this is not true.  A 'pie pumpkin' is much smaller than those set out at Halloween time.  If you visit a pumpkin patch, look for the runts that no one wants to display.

You will want to cook the pumpkin in its shell (minus the seeds and strings), so wash your pumpkin thoroughly with soap and water.

Always cook your chopped up pumpkin in a little bit of water.  ½ inch to 1 inch of water in the bottom is plenty.

After 4 hours of slow cooking, the outer shell will become separated from the meat.  If this is not the case, it needs to cook longer.

Remove the pumpkin pieces and allow to cool.  Then simply pull off the outer peel and puree the meat chunks.

Add 2 cups puree to a freezer bag, mark and store in the freezer.

The taste of genuine pumpkin is amazing and so simple

to make that you'll find yourself buying more pumpkins each year.

# Chapter 3: Making Bread

You probably never realized it, but your crock pot is a bread maker in disguise. Making your own bread can be much healthier than buying at a store, but just like all fresh foods, must be consumed quicker, due to no preservatives. While you still have to do the prep work that is required to get a loaf ready to bake, nothing tastes better than fresh, natural baked bread, right out of the oven.

Here is all the information you need to start you own bread making, and even a yummy recipe for Monkey Bread at the end.

## How to Make Sourdough Starter

Sourdough is a favorite type of dough that is used for a variety of baking, plus it is not that difficult to make. From biscuits to cakes and dumplings, sourdough just naturally tastes good. Keep your recipe close, even though you will have it memorized before long. Keep a space designated for 'growing' your first batch, as it will take 5 days to age. By using pineapple, or orange juice, there will be less cause of bad bacteria to grow.

INGREDIENTS:

5 cups flour (wheat, white or rye)

1 ¼ cups pineapple juice, room temperature
1 ½ cups water, room temperature

INSTRUCTIONS:

Day 1:  Combine 1 cup flour with ¾ cup pineapple juice in a medium sized bowl.  Whisk together and pour into a glass container, like a Mason jar.  Cover the top with a paper towel or cheesecloth and bind with a rubber band. Stir the contents in the jar twice daily.

Day 2:  Remove the contents of the jar to a medium sized bowl.  Wipe out the inside of the glass container. Add 1 cup flour and ½ cup pineapple juice to the contents and whisk.  Return to the glass jar and cover again.  Stir the contents in the jar twice daily.

Day 3:  Remove the contents of the jar to a medium sized bowl.  Remove ½ of the starter to another container and seal.  Wipe out the inside of the glass container.  This extra can be thrown out, saved as a second starter, or given to a friend.  Add 1 cup flour and ½ cup water to the contents in the bowl and whisk. Return to the glass jar and cover again.  Stir the contents in the jar twice daily.

Day 4:  Repeat Day 3, except, do not remove any more of the starter for discard.

Day 5:  Repeat Day 4.

Your starter should now show signs of fermentation with

growth and bubbles.  You can either begin the bread making process, or store in an air-tight container for up to 30 days in the refrigerator.

## How to Make Crockpot Sourdough Bread

Remove 1 cup of the starter and mix with 5 cups of flour and 2 ¼ teaspoons of salt, in a large mixing bowl.  Add up to 1 ½ cups water to create a springy, well-formed texture.

Grease the interior of your slow cooker with olive oil.

Place the mound of dough in the bottom of the crock pot and cover with a paper towel to absorb the excess moisture.  Cook for 2 hours, then check the bread and remove the paper towel.  Cook longer until desired results are reached.

## Classic Monkey Bread-Crockpot Style

Everyone loves the sweet gooey pull-apart bread that fills your nostrils with  a sugary-cinnamon scent and further, delights the taste buds.  A warm sour bread dough, baked to perfection, is one of the simple creations you can make from your sourdough starter. The smiles that this bread will bring, is worth the anticipation of feeding your new project for 5 days.

INGREDIENTS:

12 rolls of dough, biscuit size
½ cup sugar
½ cup dark sugar
4 teaspoons cinnamon
8 ounces melted butter

INSTRUCTIONS:

Line a crock pot with parchment so it rises along the sides about an inch.

Spray the interior of the crock pot with canola oil.

In a medium-sized bowl, mix the sugars and cinnamon. Place the melted butter in a separate bowl. Take each ball of dough and cut into fourths.

Dredge each piece of dough through the butter, then roll in the sugar mixture.

Place each dough piece in a circle until the entire bottom is covered with small sugar-coated balls. Cover with a piece of paper towel so the condensation will not drip on the tops.

Cover and cook for 2-3 hours. Simply lift out the parchment and serve.

# Chapter 4: Quick and Easy Breakfast Recipes

## Cinnamon Laced Oatmeal

Makes 6 Servings

Pure rolled oats make the best oatmeal, in a crock pot. Low gluten and no additives make all the difference in your choice of oats.  Because oatmeal can have a bland flavor, this crock pot recipe dresses up the flavor with applesauce, cinnamon and nutmeg.  Allowed to blend and simmer with these wonderful ingredients, you will not need a ton of brown sugar to enjoy the taste.

INGREDIENTS:

1 ½  cups pure rolled oats
1 ½  cups milk
5 cups water
¼  cup natural sugar substitute
½  cup unsweetened applesauce
1 ½  TBSP cinnamon
½  tsp nutmeg
½  tsp salt
1 tsp vanilla

INSTRUCTIONS:

Using canola oil, spray a light coat of oil on the inside of the crock pot.

Mix the liquid ingredients together, along with the rolled oats, in the crock pot. Add the applesauce, sugar substitute, cinnamon, nutmeg, salt and vanilla and stir.

Turn on the crock pot and put in a good 8 hours sleep. Upon rising your oatmeal will be ready to eat and your home, filled with the cinnamon aroma.

# Oscar Benedict Casserole

Makes 6 Servings

A variation of Eggs Benedict, an Australian favorite, this crock pot casserole gives you the rich sauce of smooth cheeses, wrapped around the succulent flavors of asparagus and crab meat.  This will make a special breakfast on a Sunday or holiday to start off a great day.

INGREDIENTS

12 hard-boiled eggs, chopped
½ cup fresh asparagus cuts
½ cup crab meat, shredded
¼ cup fresh sliced mushrooms
4 TBSP butter
1 cup milk
8 ounces cream cheese
1 small onion, chopped
1 10-1/2 ounce container cream of mushroom soup
6 English muffins

INSTRUCTIONS

Spray the interior of the crock pot with Canola oil.

In the slow cooker, combine butter, cream cheese, onion, milk and chicken soup.  Slow cook for 2 hours, then stir. Add the eggs, asparagus cuts, mushrooms, and crab meat.  Allow to cook for 6-8 hours.

Toast the English muffins and pour on the sauce.

# Yummy French Toast

Makes 6 Servings

Weekends are a time for relaxing and making special treats for the family.  Waking to the scent of cinnamon and knowing that French toast awaits you, is the perfect way to begin the day.  Simple to assemble the night before, you will find your breakfast ready to eat.

INGREDIENTS:

½ loaf bread (white, Italian, or cinnamon raisin)
6 eggs
2 cups milk
1 TBSP brown sugar
1 teaspoon vanilla

INSTRUCTIONS:

Spray the interior of the crock pot with canola oil.

In a large mixing bowl, combine the eggs, milk, sugar and vanilla.  Beat to a smooth consistency.

Dip each piece of bread in the egg mixture and place, scattered, in the crock pot.  Pour any extra batter on top.

Cover and cook for 6 to 7 hours.  Turn off crock pot, remove lid, and allow to cool for 15 minutes.

Remove and serve with maple syrup.

# Lemon-Drizzled Blueberry Pancakes

Makes 4 Servings

Surprisingly moist and flavorful pancakes can be made in your crock pot where none of the natural flavors are allowed to escape.  The secret is in this special batter, designed for slow cooking.  Your family will be amazed at your ability to turn this long-time favorite into a must have for breakfast.

INGREDIENTS

For the Batter:

1 ¼ cup flour
1/8 cup sugar
1 TBSP baking powder
½ teaspoon salt
1 egg
1 ¼ cup milk
¼ cup Canola oil
½ cup fresh blueberries

For the Glaze:

1 ½ teaspoon lemon juice
1 ½ teaspoon milk
½ cup powdered sugar

INSTRUCTIONS:

To make the batter, combine flour, sugar, baking powder and salt in a medium-sized bowl.

In a separate mixing bowl, add eggs, milk and oil. Whisk well. Pour into the dry ingredients and blend.

Place a circular piece of parchment paper in the bottom of the crock pot and spray with Canola oil.

Pour 1 cup of batter on the parchment paper. Sprinkle with blueberries. Add remaining batter on top of the blueberries.

Cover and slow cook for at least 1 hour. Test doneness with a toothpick through the center.

While your pancake is cooking, make the glaze by adding all of the ingredients and blending until smooth.

When your pancake is done, remove, drizzle with the glaze, and cut into 4 serving pieces. Pass the maple syrup, if desired.

# Crock Pot Creamy Grits

Warm your body with soothing Southern grits, keeping you feel satisfied all morning.  This recipe takes a nutritious grain and turns it into an appealing, appetizing breakfast meal.  Great for a planned morning of hiking, bicycle riding or any type of outdoor activity.

Makes 4 Servings

INGREDIENTS:

1 cup stone-ground grits
2 cups water
1 ½ cup milk
½ cup heavy cream
1 teaspoon salt
1 TBSP butter

INSTRUCTIONS:

Grease an oven-proof, 4-cup container with the butter.

In the container, combine the grits, milk, cream and salt.

Place the bowl in the crock pot and pour enough water in the bottom of the crock pot to cover up to ½ the sides of the container.

Slow cook for 7-8 hours.  Remove and stir.

Cheesy Hash Brown Casserole

Makes 6 Servings

Keep your hungry meat and potato crew happy with this great tasting breakfast meal, featuring hash browns and cheese.  Chicken pieces and mushrooms make it substantial in taste and texture.

1 16-ounce package frozen hash brown potatoes
8 ounces cooked chicken, diced
1 cup shredded cheddar cheese
1 bell pepper, diced
8 ounces fresh mushrooms, sliced
1 cup milk
12 eggs
6 scallions, diced
1 teaspoon salt
½ teaspoon pepper
½ garlic clove, minced
½ teaspoon paprika
½ teaspoon dry mustard

INSTRUCTIONS:

Using spray Canola oil, put a light coating on the inside of the crock pot.

Place 1/3 of the potatoes, bell peppers, onions, mushrooms, and chicken in the crock pot.  Sprinkle with 1/3 of the shredded cheese.  Repeat 2 more times.

Using a large mixing bowl, combine eggs, milk, salt, pepper, paprika, garlic powder and dry mustard. Whisk all together until smooth. Pour over the potato mixture.

Cover and cook on low for 6-8 hours.

Dish out when eggs are completely cooked.

# Sweet Grain Morning Cereal

Makes 4 Servings

This is a different type of warm cereal that gets away from the routine rolled oats or cream of wheat. By combining the best of many types of grain, you will find yourself savoring every bite. Sweetened with natural coconut, the taste is perfect and an all-morning satisfaction, filled.

INGREDIENTS:

¼ cup cracked wheat
¼ cup steel cut oats
¼ cup pearl barley
¼ cup brown rice
¼ cup coconut
3 cups water

INSTRUCTIONS:

Mix all ingredients in a crock pot and cook for 7 to 8 hours on low.

Spoon out and serve with cinnamon.

# Chapter 5: Make Ahead Lunch Time Meals

## Fruity Greek Yogurt

*Makes 8 Servings*

Just like making bread, you can start your own yogurt by using a store bought  container of all natural plain Greek yogurt.  After making one batch, you'll have your own starter for future batches.  Have plenty of small serving size cups with lids, on hand, to refrigerate.  You might want to double the quantities once your family tries this fruity, nutritional treat.

4 cups milk
¼ cup starter yogurt (all natural regular plain or Greek yogurt)
fruit

INSTRUCTIONS:

Add milk to crock pot and set on low heat for 2 ½ to 3 hours.

Turn off the unit and allow to stand for 3 hours, undisturbed.  After 3 hours, dip out 1 cup of the milk and pour into a bowl.  Mix together with the yogurt and return all to the crock pot. Do not turn the crock pot on but cover with a large towel to form an insulating blanket around the unit. Allow to set for 8 hours.

Remove ½ cup of the mixture as your next starter, seal and store.

Pour the yogurt over cheesecloth to remove excess liquid, then add the fruit of your choice. Blend well and spoon into individual containers.

# Chicken Mango with Tortilla Chips

Makes 4 Servings

The fresh, sweet taste of mangoes fill this chicken dish with a tangy flavor. Easy to make ahead and easy to grab on your way to work, your co-workers will think you stopped at a Mexican Restaurant. Either prepare the night before and place in single serving containers, or make on the weekend and freeze in freezer bags.

INGREDIENTS:

4 boneless, skinned chicken breasts
10 ounces fresh or frozen corn
1 can black beans, drained and rinsed
3 cups mango salsa
½ teaspoon lemon pepper

INSTRUCTIONS:

Place the chicken breasts in a crock pot. In a mixing bowl, mix together the corn, black beans, salsa and lemon pepper. Pour over the chicken and cook on high for 4-6 hours.

Shred the chicken with a fork before storing. Serve with tortilla chips.

# Slow Cooked Asian Noodle Bowl

Makes 6 Servings

Asian slow cooking has been a tradition for centuries with soups and sauces that capture amazing flavor in every bite. Try this recipe that uses ingredients that are responsible for this tantalizing taste. A bit of prep work is required, but well worth it for a great luncheon.

INGREDIENTS:

1 pound boneless, chicken breast, cut into small pieces
1 cup fresh carrots, sliced
1 cup onion, sliced
¼ cup fresh mushrooms, sliced
1 TBSP soy sauce
1 TBSP rice vinegar
1 teaspoon grated ginger
¼ teaspoon pepper
6 cups chicken broth, homemade
½ pounds snow peas
3 ounces soba noodles

INSTRUCTIONS:

Using your slow cooker, add chicken, carrots, onion, mushrooms, soy sauce, vinegar, ginger, pepper and chicken broth. Cook on high setting for 3 hours.

Cook the soba noodles in water on the stove top, drain

and set to the side to cool.

If you are going to freeze for later use, turn off the crock pot and add snow peas before cooling and placing in freezer bags.  If you are going to serve right away, add the snow peas 15 minutes before soup has finished cooking.  Keep the noodles in a separate package until ready to eat.

# BBQ Beef on Bun

Makes 12 Servings

Sometimes a quick sandwich is all you can afford in the middle of the day.  Have this fresh barbeque beef ready to warm up for a nutritious lunch.  There will be plenty to freeze for quick meals or to enjoy throughout the week.

INGREDIENTS:

3 pound roast, sliced to fit crock pot
2 teaspoons salt
2 cloves garlic, pressed
10 ounces beef broth
1 cup ketchup
½ cup packed brown sugar
½ cup lemon juice
3 TBSP steak sauce
1 teaspoon pepper
1 teaspoon Worcestershire sauce

INSTRUCTIONS:

Place the beef in the bottom of the crock pot.  Sprinkle with 1 teaspoon salt.

In a mixing bowl, combine the remaining salt, garlic, broth, ketchup, brown sugar, lemon juice, steak sauce, pepper and Worcestershire sauce.  Blend together, then pour over the roast.

Cover and cook on high setting for 7 hours.

When completed, tear the meat apart and pack all in freezer bags.

Thaw, rewarm and serve on buns with dill pickles and celery sticks.

# Slow-Cooker Spinach and Ricotta Lasagna

Makes 6 Servings

Lasagna has never tastes so good as when all of the flavors are allowed to blend together, forming a mouth-watering taste in each bite.  This recipe is easy to make, healthy, and can be used for lunch or dinner.  Cook it up, freeze in portions, and grab a great tasting entree instead of a noon-time burger.

INGREDINTS:

2 10 ounce packages chopped frozen spinach, thawed and drained
1 cup ricotta cheese
3 ounces grated Parmesan cheese
3 cups marinara sauce
6 lasagna noodles
6 ounces grated mozzarella cheese
½ cup water

INSTRUCTIONS:

Using a large mixing bowl, add the spinach, ricotta cheese and 2 ounces of the Parmesan cheese.  In a separate medium-sized bowl, blend together the marinara sauce and ½ cup water.

Measure ¾ cup of the marinara sauce mixture and pour in the bottom of a slow cooker.  Take 2 lasagna noodles, break to fit, and lay on top of the sauce. Add another ¾ cup of the marinara sauce and next, ½ of the spinach mixture. Top with 3 ounces of the mozzarella cheese.

Repeat this procedure. Finish by adding the remaining noodles, marinara mixture and cheeses.

Cook on low for 4 hours.

When finished, allow to cool until the lasagna can be transferred to freezer bags or dish up right away and serve with a salad.

# Home Made Chicken Nuggets

Makes 8 to 10 Servings

The price of restaurant chicken nuggets continues to increase, plus you never know how fresh the ingredients are.  Put your mind at ease by preparing your own chicken nuggets that are guaranteed fresh and delicious. Keep plenty in the freezer for hungry kids, or a nutritious lunch on the run.

INGREDIENTS:

6 boneless chicken breasts, skinned and halved
4 TBSP butter, melted
4 eggs
1 cup bread crumbs or cracker crumbs
½ teaspoon salt
½ teaspoon garlic powder

INSTRUCTIONS:

Lay out chicken breasts and cut into bite-sized pieces, about 2 inches.

Spray the interior of the crock pot with canola oil.

In a medium-sized mixing bowl, combine the butter and eggs and whisk.

Pour the crumbs into a large freezer bag, and roll over

with a rolling pin, to make extra fine crumbs.

Dip each chicken piece into the egg mixture then toss in the freezer bag to coat with the crumbs. You can add 5 or 6 pieces at a time.

Place the coated chicken pieces in the bottom of the crock pot. Do not layer but add a piece of aluminum foil on top of each layer. Poke a few holes in the foil to vent. Once all of the pieces are in the pot, further vent the pot by placing a wooden spoon or other heat resistant object between the lid and the pot.

Cook on high for 3 to 4 hours. Turn down to low until ready to serve.

# Crockpot Roast Beef Grinders

Makes 6 Servings

Now this is what you call a sandwich.  By using a loaf of Artisan Italian Bread, making slits, and stuffing with tender pieces of roast beef, cheese, and other trimmings, you can have a lunch that is fit for a king. Treat your family or co-workers with this delectable meal that puts any deli sandwich to shame.

INGREDIENTS:

1 round loaf of Artisan Italian Bread
18 thinly sliced pieces of roast beef
18 slices Mozzarella cheese
24 slices sweet pepper rings
1 onion, sliced thin
1 TBSP oregano
1 TBSP basil
¼ cup water
1 TBSP olive oil

INSTRUCTIONS:

You will need at least a 6 quart crock pot.

Begin your assembly on a cutting board by slicing the bread, evenly, into 13 sections.  Do not cut all the way through, but leave about ½ inch solid bread on the bottom of the bread.  In each slit, line with 3 pieces of roast beef.  Layer 3 slices of cheese inside of the roast beef, and top with the pepper rings and onion.  Sprinkle with the oregano and basil.

Use 2 large pieces of aluminum foil and tightly wrap the stuffed bread with 2 layers, making sure to keep the bottom crust from bowing.

Wad up 3 or 4 pieces of aluminum foil into a tight ball and place evenly in the crock pot.  Pour the water in the crock pot.   Place the stuffed bread on top of the foil balls.  This will prevent the bread from scorching.

Cook on low for 3-4 hours.  Remove and unwrap.  Drizzle the olive oil over the slits, just to add moisture.  Finish cutting all the way through the bread and serve your individual grinders.

# Chapter 6: Delightful Dinner Specialties

## Jamaican Jerk Chicken

*Makes 6 Servings*

A popular dish in the Caribbean is jerk chicken. This recipe will send your mind to the natural, sunny setting of the tropics with the tantalizing seasonings of the natives. Serve with natural greens, seasoned with coconut oil and homemade bread for a truly Jamaican experience.

INGREDIENTS:

4 pounds chicken legs
8 ounces pineapple slices
12 ounces jerk marinade
½ teaspoon garlic powder
½ teaspoon onion powder
½ teaspoon paprika
½ teaspoon allspice
2 ½ teaspoons crushed red pepper
1 teaspoon liquid smoke
¼ cup brown sugar
4 cloves garlic
1 hot pepper, seeded and chopped

nutmeg and cinnamon to taste
2 cups water

INSTRUCTIONS:

Place chicken legs in crock pot.

Add garlic powder, onion powder, paprika, allspice, red pepper, and brown sugar.  Next, add pineapple slices, liquid smoke, garlic and hot pepper.

Top with the marinade and enough water to cover all of the chicken pieces.

Cover and cook on high for 6 hours.  Taste test the sauce and add cinnamon and nutmeg for extra flavor.  Turn to low and continue cooking for another 1 to 2 hours.

# Mock Swiss Steak

Makes 6 Servings

The cost of beef may have you cutting back on favorite meats, but this is where a slow cooker can work miracles.  Take a tough round steak and transform into a replica of a mouth-watering Swiss steak that tastes like the real McCoy.  This process can also work with gamey meat and other inferior cuts of beef.

INGREDIENTS:

2 pounds round steak
4 TBSP cornstarch or potato starch
1 TBSP butter
1 chopped onion
1 16-ounce can chopped tomatoes with green chilies
3 cloves garlic
2 TBSP liquid aminos
1 ¼ cup water

INSTRUCTIONS:

Cut steak into 6 serving sizes.  Tenderize each piece by pounding with a mallet.  Place the starch on a plate and dredge the meat through to coat.

Using a skillet, melt the butter over medium heat and brown the meat.  Remove and place in the crock pot.

Brown the onions in the same skillet until almost tender, remove and add to the crock pot. Add the liquid aminos to the skillet, cook for a few seconds and pour the rest of the remaining skillet drippings to the crock pot.

Using a medium-sized bowl, combine the tomatoes, water and garlic. Blend well and pour over the contents in the crock pot.

Cover and cook on low for 8 to 10 hours.

Remove and serve over rice or noodles.

# Slow-Cooker Sesame Chicken

Makes 4 Servings

This favorite Chinese dish is sweet, tangy, and nutritional.  The whole family will love the way that honey spins great taste and pure goodness to chicken pieces.  Double the recipe and have leftovers for lunch the next day or freeze for a second meal.

INGREDIENTS:

4 chicken breasts, deboned
½ cup diced onion
2 cloves garlic, minced
½ cup honey
¼ cup ketchup
½ cup soy sauce
2 TBSP olive oil
¼ teaspoon pepper flakes
4 teaspoons cornstarch
1/3 cup water
3 scallions
1 TBSP sesame seeds
salt and pepper

INSTRUCTIONS:

Put chicken breasts in crock pot and sprinkle with salt and pepper.

Using a medium-sized mixing bowl, combine onion, garlic, ketchup, honey, soy sauce, oil, and pepper flakes. Blend and pour over chicken. Cover crock pot and cook on low for 4 hours.

Lift chicken from the pot and place on board to shred into bite-sized pieces. Cover to keep warm.

Using a small bowl, add cornstarch together with 1/3 cup water and stir. Add to sauce in the crock pot and allow to cook for 15 minutes, or until sauce begins to thicken.

Serve sauce over cooked rice, adding chicken on top. Sprinkle with scallions and sesame seeds.

# Nihari (Pakistani Beef Curry)

Makes 6 Servings

Cultural foods are becoming popular in American society.  The crock pot is a great way to prepare this old world Indian favorite, that is centuries old.  Using additives to simmer this traditional dish, shows you how natural seasonings can really wake up a beef brisket.

INGREDIENTS:

2 yellow onions, peeled and sliced
2 pounds beef brisket, fat trimmed off
1 ginger root, approximately 2 inches long, peeled and cut into chunks
10 cloves garlic, peeled and diced
1 teaspoon ground ginger
4 white cardamom pods
3 bay leaves
1 TBSP garam masala
2 TBSP ground fennel
1 TBSP ground chili pepper
1 teaspoon turmeric
2 teaspoons salt
1 teaspoon nutmeg
½ cup Canola oil

INSTRUCTIONS:

Put onions in crock pot.  Add beef brisket.

Grind the ginger and garlic to a paste and add on top of the meat.

Add all other ingredients, ending with the Canola oil being poured evenly over all.

Cook on low for 4 hours.  Turn the beef brisket over and continue cooking for an additional 4-5 hours.  Remove the brisket and shred.  Add the meat back to the sauce and toss until mixed well.

Serve over brown or basmati rice.

# Korean Beef Stew with Cabbage

Makes 6 Servings

This version of beef stew is popular in the far east, as well as many American homes.  Pickles, bean sprouts and cabbage make an exciting taste to this internationally acclaimed dish.  This will take a bit longer than most slow cooker recipe but the results are amazing.

INGREDIENTS:

1 TBSP Canola oil
3 pounds beef chuck
¼ cup soy sauce
¼ cup sugar
1 quart beef stock
2 red onions, peeled and quartered
6 cloves garlic, peeled and chopped
1 jalapeno peppers, seeded and chopped
2 cups bean sprouts
1 TBSP cornstarch
4 cups Napa cabbage
½ cup sliced dill pickles
2 TBSP scallions
Sesame seed oil


INSTRUCTIONS:

Start with a large skillet on the stove top. Add the Canola oil and warm over medium-high heat. Add the meat and sear until brown on both sides. Remove the meat and place in the crock pot. Cover and turn on high.

Using the same skillet, pour out any remaining oil and wipe clean. Place back on burner and stock, soy sauce, and sugar. Heat to boiling, then add to meat in the crock pot. Add onions and cover. Cook for 2 hours on high.

Remove lid after 2 hours and add garlic and jalapenos. Cover and continue cooking for an additional 1 hour.

In a small bowl, mix the cornstarch with ½ cup of stew juices.

Remove the meat and place on a board for shredding. Remove the onions and discard. Whisk the cornstarch mixture with the crock pot drippings and cover the pot.

Turn crock pot on low and allow to simmer for a few minutes. Next, add the shredded meat back to the pot and stir until coated with the sauce.

In a medium-sized saucepan, bring 2 cups of water to a boil. Add the bean sprouts and blanch for 30 seconds. Remove from heat, drain and set to the side.

Add the cabbage and pickles to the crock pot, without disturbing the other ingredients, and cover. Cook until the cabbage is wilted, about 5 minutes. Turn off the cooker.

Prepare steamed rice and spoon the stew over. Top with bean sprouts, scallions, and drizzle sesame oil over all.

# Saucy Slow Cooker Meatballs

Makes 6 Servings

Meatballs can make a variety of dishes. Use to add zest to pasta, make hoagie sandwiches, or serve as a main dish along with a side or two. The robust flavor of tomatoes and beef creates a hearty meal, with little time. This recipe can be made up to 2 days in advance and refrigerated.

INGREDIENTS:

2 28-ounce cans whole tomatoes, or fresh peeled
2 TBSP olive oil
2 TBSP tomato paste
1 sprig basil
¼ teaspoon red pepper
4 garlic cloves, minced
2 pounds ground chuck beef
3 TBSP dry bread crumbs
1 egg, beaten
3 TBSP grated Parmesan cheese
1 TBSP salt
¼ teaspoon pepper

INSTRUCTIONS;

Place the whole tomatoes in the bottom of the crock pot, then squish them down with the back of a ladle or a gloved palm. If using canned tomatoes, empty the remaining juice on top.

Add ½ of the garlic, olive oil, tomato paste, basil, and red pepper. Place the cover on the pot and cook for 3 hours on high.

Take a large mixing bowl, while the sauce is cooking, and add the remaining garlic, ground chuck, bread crumbs, egg, Parmesan cheese, salt and pepper.
Mix well and form into small balls. You should be able to make 18 to 20 balls.

When the sauce has reached 3 hours of cooking, add the meatballs. Cover and cook on high for an additional 1 to 2 hours. Carefully remove the meatballs, pour a generous portion of sauce over, and serve.

# Chapter 7: Favorite Slow Cooking Recipes for Crowds

## Crock Pot Chicken Fajitas

Makes 8 Servings

Forget the hamburgers and hot dogs at your next party and give your guests a hearty meal that will rate as number 1.  This recipe for chicken fajitas is easy to prepare, healthy, and a great change from the norm.  Let your slow cooker do all the work and lay out your spread, when the time is right.  Double the recipe for extra visitors or put some back for another day.

INGREDIENTS:

2 red bell peppers, quartered and sliced
2 green bell peppers, quartered and sliced
1 large diced onion
2 ½ cups of your favorite salsa
2 TBSP flour
2 packages fajita seasoning mix
2 pounds skinless chicken breast (raw), cut into strips
flour tortillas
sour cream

INSTRUCTIONS:

On a cutting board, slice the chicken into thin 2-inch strips.

In a small mixing bowl, mix the fajita seasoning and flour together. Coat the chicken strips with this mixture and add to the crock pot.

Add onions and salsa, cover and cook for 6-8 hours on low.

Dip out the chicken and sauce into a large serving bowl and surround with a bowl of the bell peppers, flour tortillas and sour cream.

# Gourmet Macaroni and Cheese

Makes 12 Servings

This dish will be the first the disappear once word gets around to 'try the macaroni and cheese'. Four savory cheeses and evaporated milk makes this the tastiest dish on the table. It doesn't matter if the weather is warm or cold, good taste is always popular.

INGREDIENTS:

½ pound elbow macaroni
2 TBSP butter
2 TBSP flour
2 cups milk
½ TBSP Worcestershire sauce
½ teaspoon dry mustard
½ teaspoon salt
½ teaspoon pepper
6 ounces Cheddar cheese, shredded
4 ounces Gruyere cheese, shredded
4 ounces mozzarella cheese, shredded
1 ounce fresh Parmesan cheese, grated
3 fresh diced tomatoes
½ cup breadcrumbs

INSTRUCTIONS:

On the stove top, boil macaroni in water until al dente, about 5 to 7 minutes. Drain, rinse and set aside.

In another medium-sized saucepan, melt the butter. Add the flour and stir until blended. Add the milk and continue stirring until the sauce comes to a boil. Stir in Worcestershire sauce and dry mustard. Turn off heat and add the Cheddar and Gruyere cheeses. Stir until melted. Add the macaroni and stir until coated.

Prepare the crock pot by spraying the interior with Canola oil. Add ½ of the macaroni mixture, then add the diced tomatoes. Layer the mozzarella cheese on the tomatoes, then top with the rest of the macaroni.

Mix breadcrumbs and ½ of the Parmesan cheese together and sprinkle on top.

Cook on low for 5-6 hours. Remove and sprinkle with remaining Parmesan cheese.

# Crowd Pleasing BBQ Beef Ribs

Makes 8-10 Servings

BBQ Beef Ribs are great for a cook-out but no one wants to spend the day watching the meat. Cure this problem by slow cooking your meal the night before and still offer the same tantalizing flavor of smoky, moist ribs. Keep in the crock pot or lay out on the grill for 30 or 40 minutes before serving. The crowd will be in awe at the tender, flavor-rich meat.

INGREDIENTS:

4 pounds boneless beef short ribs
2 cups water
1 18-ounce bottle barbeque sauce
1 TBSP Worcestershire sauce
3 ounces hickory smoke sauce
¼ teaspoon angostura
¼ TBSP lemon pepper

INSTRUCTIONS:

Place all ingredients in the crock pot, cover, and cook on low for 12 hours.

# Garden Fresh Chunky Pasta Sauce

Makes 12 Servings

Not sure of the number of people that you will be serving?  Make this heavenly fresh sauce with leftovers from the garden and bring out, as needed.  Tomatoes, pepper, squash and onions in a delectable creamy sauce, will impress your guests and family.  Boil up the pasta, as needed, and spread on this incredible sauce.  Make ahead of time and refrigerate, then heat as needed.

INGREDIENTS:

6 large fresh tomatoes, cut into chunks
2 green peppers, diced
1 zucchini or yellow squash, grated
2 carrots, peeled and grated
16 garlic cloves, minced
2 cups onions, diced
2 bay leaves
2 teaspoons oregano
2 TBSP dried oregano
2 TBSP tomato paste
2 TBSP quick cooking tapioca
2 TBSP basil, fresh or dried
2 teaspoons salt
1 teaspoon pepper
2 TBSP Canola oil

Combine the onion and Canola oil in a bowl and microwave for 3 to 4 minutes, stirring a couple of times.

In a crock pot, add the tomatoes, peppers, squash, garlic, carrots, tomato paste and tapioca. Pour the onions on top.

Cover and cook on high for 4 hours, or low for 8 hours.

Serve or measure into air tight containers for later.

# Tangy Honey Chicken Wings

Makes 12 Servings

Chicken wings are a favorite at any type of gathering. Make these simple tangy wings that are sure to be a hit. Real honey, garlic and lots of slow cooking will deliver a mouth-watering extravaganza. Perfect for feeding hungry teens or snacking on during your favorite sports game.

INGREDIENTS:

30-40 chicken wings (about 3 pounds)
¾ cup honey
1 ½ TBSP minced garlic
2 TBSP olive oil
½ teaspoon salt
½ teaspoon pepper

INSTRUCTIONS:

In a medium-sized bowl, mix the honey, olive oil, garlic, salt and pepper.

Put the chicken wings in the crock pot and pour the honey mixture over all.

Cook on low for 6 hours.

Remove and serve.

# Zesty Crock Pot Chili

Makes 10 Servings

Nothing goes over as well as a big pot of chili. Make this recipe that delivers a zesty and spicy meal for a hungry crowd. This is a thick recipe that can be thinned down by adding water or tomato juice to your liking.

INGREDIENTS:

2 pounds ground beef
1 cup onion, chopped
1 TBSP minced garlic
½ cup celery, chopped
2 15-ounce cans diced tomatoes
1 15-ounce can tomato sauce
1 15-ounce can pinto beans
1 15-ounce can red kidney beans
4 TBSP chili powder
1 TBSP cumin
1 teaspoon paprika
1 teaspoon chipotle powder
water or tomato juice for thinning

INSTRUCTIONS:

Using a large skillet, brown the ground beef, along with the onion and garlic over medium-high heat. Add the celery and continue cooking until the meat is cooked throughout. Turn off the stove and remove the grease drippings.

In the crock pot, add the tomatoes, tomato sauce, pinto beans, red kidney beans, chili powder, cumin, paprika and chipotle powder. Add the hamburger mixture. Stir and add water or tomato juice to the consistency desired. Cover and cook on low for 8 hours.

Remove lid and stir. If the chili is still too thick for your liking, add more liquid and continue cooking for an additional hour.

# Chapter 8: Awesome Soups

## Flavorful Chicken Noodle Soup

Makes 6 Servings

Everyone loves the warmth and soothing flavor that chicken soup brings. Packed full of fresh vegetables and homemade chicken broth, this recipe will disappear quickly. Always keep extra chicken broth on hand to make your next batch, when requested.

INGREDIENTS:

5 cups homemade chicken broth
1 can cream of chicken soup
½ cup onion, finely chopped
½ cup celery, finely chopped
½ cup carrots, finely chopped
½ cup sliced green onions
1 cup fresh corn
2 cups cooked, chopped chicken
1 ½ cup egg noodles

INSTRUCTIONS:

In a slow cooker, add the chicken broth, soup, onion, celery, carrots, green onions and corn. Cook on low for 5 hours.

Dip out and serve.

# French Potato Leek Soup

Makes 6 Servings

If you have ever heard of Julia Child, you understand how good French cooking can leave you hooked on the awesome flavor. One of her favorite starter recipes for young cooks was this simple, yet rich and hearty soup, that fills your senses with the prestigious dishes of France. So elementary to learn and remember, you will make regularly.

INGREDIENTS:

4 medium-sized leeks, using the white part only, and sliced thin

4 large russet potatoes, peeled and diced

5 to 6 cups vegetable or chicken stock

2 TBSP butter

INSTRUCTIONS:

Place the leeks and potatoes in a crock pot and cover with just enough stock to cover the vegetables.

Cook on low for 7 hours.

Turn off the crock pot and use an immersion blender on

the soup, or dip out in batches and puree in a food processor. Add a pinch of salt, if needed, and blend in the butter.

Pour into bowls and serve with warm French bread.

# Classic Oxtail Soup

Makes 6 Servings

If you have never experienced the taste of oxtail soup, you are missing a special treat. There is no way to describe the taste of oxtail, except to say that it is the best beef you have ever had. Try this classic recipe that combines flavor-rich oxtail meat with spices and vegetables. Lentils or beans can also be used.

INGREDIENTS:

4 pounds disjointed oxtails
3 TBSP olive oil
2 onions, chopped
2 garlic cloves, minced
1 TBSP flour
2 cups beef stock
1 cup tomato sauce
6 peppercorns
½ teaspoon oregano
1 red chili pepper, seeded and chopped
2 cloves
2 carrots, chopped
1 red bell pepper, chopped
1 TBSP parsley, chopped
2 potatoes, cut into chucks
salt and pepper

INSTRUCTIONS:

Using a large skillet, warm the olive oil and add the oxtails. Brown on all sides over medium-high heat. Add the garlic and onion and cook for 5 minutes. Sprinkle the flour over the meat and stir all for 2 minutes. Turn off the stove.

In the crock pot, add the potatoes in the bottom and add the meat and drippings. Next, add the carrots, then the remaining ingredients.

Cover and cook on low for 9 to 11 hours.

Remove meat and vegetables with a slotted spoon and pour the soup on top. Serve with homemade bread.

# Creamy Broccoli Cheese Soup

Makes 4 Servings

Tasty, creamy, warm and filling, this recipe for broccoli cheese soup is always a favorite. The cream, chicken stock, and fresh vegetables make this dish a favorite for all ages. You will swear that it is better than any 5-star restaurant serves.

INGREDIENTS:

1 TBSP butter
½ onion, chopped
¼ cup melted butter
¼ cup flour
2 cups half-and-half
2 cups chicken stock
½ pound fresh broccoli
1 cup carrot, cut in julienne strips
¼ teaspoon nutmeg
8 ounces sharp cheddar cheese, cubed

INSTRUCTIONS:

In a crock pot, melt the 1 tablespoon butter and stir in the onion with the pot set on high. Add the flour and ¼ cup melted butter and stir.

Add 1 cup of the half-and-half and stir until smooth. Add the other cup and stir.

Pour in the broccoli and chicken stock and blend well. Add the nutmeg and carrot.

Put the lid on the crock pot and turn the heat to low. Cook for 6 hours. Remove the lid and add the cheese. Cook for an additional hour. Turn off crock pot and stir all contents until creamy.

Remove and serve.

# Crock Pot Tomato Soup

Makes 4 Servings

Use fresh from the garden tomatoes and chicken stock to create a smooth tasting soup.  The natural ingredients will make you feel satisfied without having  a heavy, after meal feeling.  Great for lunch time or as a side with sandwiches.

INGREDIENTS:

2 TBSP butter
¼ cup onion
6 cups chopped tomatoes
1 ½ cup chicken stock
1 teaspoon salt
1 cup heavy cream

INSTRUCTIONS:

Using a small skillet, sauté the onions in butter.  Add to crock pot.

Place chicken stock and tomatoes on top of the onions. Cover and cook on low for 6 hours.

Turn off crock pot and puree with the heavy cream by either using an immersion blender or a regular blender. If a stand up blender is used, puree in batches of 2 cups, or less.

Transfer to bowls and sprinkle with salt for desired taste.

# Chapter 9: Delicious Desserts

## Sweet Potato Pudding Cake

Makes 8 Servings

As more and more people are discovering the health benefits of sweet potatoes,
recipes are abounding.  This delightful dessert uses coconuts and pecans to add a sweet flavor to this vegetable that is starting to turn heads with popularity.

INGREDIENTS:

½ cup butter
2 cups flour
1 teaspoon baking powder
½ teaspoon baking soda
¼ teaspoon salt
2 teaspoons cinnamon
1 cup brown sugar
1 1-ounce can sweet potatoes, drained
2 eggs
2 teaspoons vanilla extract
¾ cup coconut milkshakes1/2 cup pecans, chopped
¼ cup flaked coconut, toasted
1 cup dulce de leche

INSTRUCTIONS:

Using a small sauce pan, melt the butter over medium heat. Whisk until it begins to turn a brownish color. Remove from heat and pour into a large mixing bowl.

In a medium-sized mixing bowl, combine the flour, baking powder, baking soda, salt and cinnamon. Mix.

Mash sweet potatoes and add to the bowl of butter. Add brown sugar and beat together with an electric mixer. When creamy, add the eggs and vanilla and beat well.

Turn mixer speed to low and gradually add flour mixture, pouring in the coconut milk to keep moist. Continue mixing until smooth. Stir in pecans.

Spray the inside of the crock pot with canola oil and add the batter. Cover and cook for 45 minutes on low.

Remove lid and add the dulce de leche on top, spreading out evenly. Sprinkle with the toasted coconut and cover. Bake for 1 hour. Turn off the crock pot and allow to absorb the flavors for 45 minutes.

# Apple Filled Coffee Cake

Makes 8 Servings

Whoever heard of baking a cake in a crock pot? It's easier than you think and keeps the texture moist and full of flavor. Weave in your favorite fruits for a wonderful flavor that will need no icing.

INGREDIENTS:

1 20-ounce can apple pie filling
1 teaspoon cinnamon
3 TBSP brown sugar
2 9-ounce yellow cake mixes
2 eggs, beaten
½ cup sour cream
3 TBSP butter, melted
½ cup evaporated milk

INSTRUCTIONS:

In a medium-sized bowl, combine pie filling, brown sugar, and ½ teaspoon cinnamon.

Using a separate medium-sized bowl, add the cake mixes, eggs, sour cream, butter and milk. Mix well.

Spray the interior of the crock pot with canola oil.

Spread ½ of the apple mixture in the bottom of the crock

pot.  Pour ½ of the batter on top.

Add the remaining apple mixture, then the rest of the batter.

Cover and cook on high for 2 hours.  Test with a toothpick for doneness.  If needed, continue cooking for an additional ½ to 1 hour.  When done, turn off the crock pot and remove the lid.

Allow to cool for 15 minutes before inverting onto a serving plate.

# Crock Pot Pumpkin Pie Treat

Makes 8 Servings

Discover how pumpkin pie can taste fresh and delicious by trying this unusual recipe. Using pumpkin puree, spices, and Bisquick, there will be no sogginess, and no store-bought artificial flavor. By slow cooking, you can also set off a heavenly scent of a hard day's baking, but with little effort.

INGREDIENTS:

1 15-ounce can pumpkin puree
9 ounces evaporated milk
¾ cup brown sugar
3 ounces maple extract
2/3 cup Bisquick
2 beaten eggs
3 TBSP butter
2 teaspoons pumpkin pie spice

INSTRUCTIONS:

Using a large mixing bowl, combine pumpkin, milk, maple extract, brown sugar and 1/3 cup of Bisquick. Mix well and pour into the crock pot. Cut the butter into pats and place on top of the mixture. Sprinkle with the remaining Bisquick.

Cook on low for 6 to 7 hours or until the mixture has

thickened and is golden brown.

Scoop out and serve with whipped cream or ice cream.

# Donut Custard Delight

Makes 12 Servings

This dessert is great for coming up with a special treat when ingredients are limited.  Grab some donuts and eggs and you're halfway there.  A smooth vanilla custard, packed full of exciting cake flavor, will delight your family and friends.

INGREDIENTS:

1 dozen donuts (yeast or cake)
½ gallon half-and-half
1 dozen eggs
½ cup sugar
1 TBSP cinnamon

INSTRUCTIONS:

Spray the interior of the crock pot with Canola oil.

In a large mixing bowl, mix the eggs, half-and-half, sugar and cinnamon.

Tear the donuts into large chunks and place in the crock pot.

Pour the half-and-half mixture over the donuts and cover.

Cook on low for 6 hours.

To add more flavor to your custard dessert, use jelly donuts of your favorite flavor.

# Chocolate Peanut Butter Cake

Makes 8 Servings

Thick, gooey chocolate and rich peanut butter flavor are the two characteristics of this yummy dessert. Crock pot friendly and simple to assemble, your cake will be a winner after dinner, as a snack, or as a carry-in dish

INGREDIENTS

1 cup flour
1 cup sugar
1 teaspoon backing powder
½ teaspoon salt
½ cup creamy peanut butter
½ cup milk
1 TBSP canola oil
1 teaspoon vanilla
3 TBSP unsweetened cocoa powder
1 cup boiling water

INSTRUCTIONS:

Spray the interior of the crock pot with canola oil. Using a mixing bowl, combine the flour, ½ cup sugar, baking powder and salt.

Place the peanut butter in a microwavable dish and microwave for 30 seconds. Pour the peanut butter into the flour batter. Stir well.

Pour the contents into the crock pot.

In a medium-sized bowl, mix the remaining sugar, cocoa powder and 1 cup of boiling water.  Stir, then pour over the contents of the crock pot.

Cover and cook on high for 3-4 hours.  Turn off the crock pot and allow to sit for 30 minutes before serving.

# Sweet Caramel Rice Pudding

Makes 8 Servings

The warm, sweet taste of homemade rice pudding just got even better with this updated version. By using condensed milk and slow cooking, caramelization takes place and leaves not only a luscious taste, but this dessert a beautiful glossy, golden color.

INGREDIENTS:

3 cups white rice, cooked
½ cup raisins
1 teaspoon vanilla
1 14-ounce can condensed milk
1 12-ounce can evaporated milk
1 TBSP sugar
1 teaspoon cinnamon

INSTRUCTIONS:

Using spray canola oil, lightly coat the inside of the crock pot.

Add all ingredients, except for the cinnamon and sugar. Mix well with a long spoon.

Cook for 3 to 4 hours, remove lid and stir. If all the liquid has been absorbed, place the pudding in bowls and sprinkle with sugar and cinnamon.

# Cherry-Apple Cobbler

Makes 8 Servings

Apples and cherries were meant for one another in this sweet and tart dessert that uses crescent rolls as crust. The thick, tapioca sauce gives a special zing to the wholesome fruit.

INGREDIENTS:

½ cup sugar
4 teaspoons quick-cooking tapioca
1 teaspoon apple spice
1 ½ pounds apples, cored, peeled and sliced
1 16-ounce can pitted cherries
½ cup dried cherries
1 package crescent roll triangles
1 TBSP sugar
½ teaspoon apple spice
1 TBSP melted butter

INSTRUCTIONS:

Add to the crock pot, the tapioca, 1 teaspoon apple spice and ½ cup sugar. Blend well. Add the apple slices and cherries, using the liquid from the can. Toss to coat with the tapioca mixture.

Cover and cook on high for 3 hours.

Warm oven to 375 degrees.

Using a small mixing bowl, add the 1 TBSP sugar, ½ teaspoon apple spice and 1 TBSP melted butter.

Unroll the crescent triangles and cut each one into thirds.  Brush each piece with the melted butter mixture.

Move coated pieces to an ungreased cookie sheet and place in the oven for 8 to 10 minutes.  Remove and cool.

Dip out the cherry-apple sauce and top with the apple spice crescent pieces.

Serve with light cream or vanilla bean ice cream.

# Chapter 10: Snacks, Drinks and More

## Warm Cinnamon Almonds

Makes 8 to 12 Servings

Move over chips and candy, because the almonds have arrived. Healthy, sweet and nutty, these treats will quickly become a weekly routine. Keep them handy on the kitchen counter where they are a welcome snack between meals. It may be wise to keep a supply in air-tight bags, just in case you run out.

INGREDIENTS:

1 ½ cups white sugar
1 ½ cups brown sugar
3 TBSP cinnamon
1/8 teaspoon salt
1 egg white
2 teaspoons vanilla
3 cups almonds
¼ cup water

INSTRUCTIONS:

Using a large bowl, mix together the white and brown sugar, salt and cinnamon.

In a separate large bowl, add the egg white and vanilla. Whisk until frothy.  Add almonds and coat thoroughly.

Spray a light coat of canola oil inside the crock pot.  Place the coated almonds inside the pot, then add the brown sugar mix.  Toss to coat.

Cook on low for 3 to 4 hours, stirring often.  During the last 30 minutes, add the water and stir.  This adds a crunchy exterior to the nuts and help to harden.

Remove onto parchment paper and carefully separate. They will be sticky and clump together but will harden further when exposed to the air.

# Spicy Pecans

Makes 8 Servings

Watch as pecans take on a new flavor when slow cooked in spices. A Cajun taste is the result by blending different seasonings and steaming to perfection. Place in a jar and give as homemade gifts next Christmas. Yes, they are that good.

INGREDIENTS:

1 pound pecan halves
¼ cup melted butter
1 teaspoon dried basil
1 teaspoon dried oregano
1 teaspoon dried thyme
½ teaspoon onion powder
¼ teaspoon garlic powder
¼ teaspoon ground cayenne pepper
1 teaspoon salt

INSTRUCTIONS:

Place all ingredients (except pecans) in a mixing bowl and blend.

Put the pecans in the crock pot. Cover with the spice mix and toss.

Place the lid on the crock pot and cook on high for 15

minutes.  Turn on low and cook for an additional 2 hours, stirring occasionally.

Remove and let cook on a cookie sheet or parchment paper.

# Beefy Taco Dip

Makes 8 Servings

Turn the ordinary into the extra-ordinary with this upbeat taco dip that is satisfying and rich in flavor. A mixture of cheese, salsa, and hamburger create a lively flavor. Be careful, however, because this dip can also be very addicting.

INGREDIENTS:

½ pound ground chuck
1 cup frozen corn
½ cup chopped onion
½ cup salsa
½ cup mild taco sauce
4 ounces mild green chilies, diced
4 ounces black olives, drained and sliced
1 cup Mexican shredded cheese

INSTRUCTIONS:

Cook the ground chuck in a skillet on the stove. Drain off the grease and put the meat in the crock pot.

Add the corn, onion, salsa, taco sauce green chilies and black olives. Stir.

Cook on low for 4 to 6 hours. Turn off the crock pot, stir in the cheese and turn into a serving bowl.

# Spicy Apricot Juice

Makes 8 Servings

Try this picker-upper instead of regular store-bought juices that are heavily laced with sugar. You know what the ingredients are and you will discover what natural flavor really means. Perfect for storing in the refrigerator or serving with any meal of the day.

INGREDIENTS:

46 ounces apricot nectar
3 cups orange juice
½ cup packed brown sugar
2 TBSP fresh lemon juice
3 sticks cinnamon
2 cloves, whole

INSTRUCTIONS:

Using your slow cooker, add orange juice, apricot nectar, brown sugar and lemon juice. Stir.

Place the cinnamon sticks and cloves in a small cheesecloth bag and tie. Add the bag to the juice.

Cook on low for 3-5 hours.

Perfect served hot on cool days or served iced, on warm days.

# Hot Chocolate Surprise

Makes 12 Servings

Spending family time outside raking leaves or decorating for the holidays will become a tradition that includes the smell of freshly made hot chocolate. Let this rich and creamy treat fill your home with memories, then enjoy the surprisingly mellow flavor.

INGREDIENTS:

3 cups dry powdered milk
1 cup powdered sugar
¾ cup cocoa powder
¼ teaspoon salt
2 teaspoons vanilla
½ cup chocolate syrup
½ cup creamer
7 cups water
Mini marshmallows
Peppermint sticks

INSTRUCTIONS:

Place the milk, sugar, cocoa, salt, vanilla, chocolate syrup and creamer in a crock pot. Stir until blended.

Gradually add water while whisking. Cover and cook on low for 4 hours. Stir before serving. Dip into mugs and add marshmallows and a peppermint stick, to use as a stirrer.

# Chocolate Fondue

Makes 2 cups for Dipping

Warm, glossy milk chocolate is the result for this simple recipe that entices everyone to dip. You can use strawberries, pineapple pieces or apples as a fruit. Angel food cake squares, pretzels or Biscotti are also favorites for dipping.

INGREDIENTS:

24 ounces semi-sweet chocolate chip pieces
1 ¼ cup evaporated milk
¼ cup sugar
2 teaspoons vanilla

INSTRUCTIONS:

Add all ingredient to a crock pot. Cover and cook on high for 30 minutes. Remove cover, stir and reduce heat to low. Cover and cook for an additional 1 hour. Remove to a smaller container or leave in the crock where the chocolate will remain warm.

# Rice Crispy Bars

Makes 12 Servings

This treat is a favorite among the kids but can be so cumbersome to make. Cut your time, and the mess back considerably, by using your crock pot as a tool. You'll be able to stop dreading the steps involved when they become simple to make.

INGREDIENTS:

3 TBSP butter, melted
4 cups miniature marshmallows or 40 regular sized
6 cups rice crispy cereal

INSTRUCTIONS:

Place the butter in the bottom of the crock pot.

Add the marshmallows then top with the cereal.

Cover and cook on high for 1 hour. Remove the lid and stir with a wooden spoon. If the marshmallows have not completely melted into a gooey mix, continue cooking for another ½ hour. Remove lid and allow to cool for 15 minutes.

Spray a 9x11 cookie sheet with canola oil. Pour the mixture onto the sheet and spread evenly. Use waxed paper to flatten the cereal to prevent the marshmallow cream from sticking to your hands.  Allow to harden for 1 hour, cut into bars, and serve.

# Chapter 11: 5-Day Meal Planner

**Day 1**

Breakfast – Crock pot Creamy Grits, Toast, Juice

Lunch -- Homemade yogurt, salad, rice pudding, sparkling water

Dinner -- Saucy meatballs over pasta, garlic bread, lemonade

**Day 2**

Breakfast -- Granola cereal, yogurt, sliced strawberries and bananas, juice

Lunch -- Asian noodle bowl, freshly made applesauce, hot green tea

Dinner -- Barbeque beef ribs, coleslaw, French bread, apple juice

**Day 3**

Breakfast -- Slow cooker pancakes, juice

Lunch -- Chicken Mango with Tortilla chips, rice pudding, green tea

Dinner -- Macaroni and Cheese, salad, sour dough bread, iced tea

## Day 4

Breakfast -- Cheesy Hash brown Casserole, toast, juice

Lunch -- Asian noodle bowl, salad, celery and carrot sticks, green tea

Dinner -- Korean Beef Stew, sour dough bread, applesauce, cherry-apple cobbler, iced tea

## Day 5

Breakfast -- Granola cereal, fresh melon, coffee or hot tea

Lunch -- Chicken Mango with Tortilla chips, donut pudding, sparkling water

Dinner -- Chicken wings, chips and salsa, fresh corn, monkey bread, milkshakes

Many of the meals that you prepare in the crock pot can be saved until the next day and have ready to warm up for lunch. The same holds true with desserts and snacks when you need something on the run.

# Conclusion to Crock Pot Cooking

All of the recipes listed are based on a 6-quart crock pot but a 4-quart will also work.  For smaller models, simply cut the ingredients in half.  Cooking time can also be decreased if the recipe notes a low setting.  Using the high setting, as opposed to the low setting, can reduce the cooking time by one-third the time.

Double or triple the ingredients for the slow cooking crowd recipes, depending on the number of guests that you have.  A larger pot will be needed, or use multiple crock pots.  You may also freeze any of these dishes and have on hand to serve for dinner when time is short.

Slow cooking can be a radical change to those that have lived their entire lives with speed and impatience.  However, once you get used to the genuine taste that great food can deliver through a crock pot, you will easily adjust your schedule.

Quicker is not always better, as we have seen in a society that is overweight and  harnesses several ailments.  This book was not designed to place you on any type of diet, but to learn the basics and assets that slow cooking can bring to your life.  You will find that there is no extra burden of time placed upon your schedule, but a simple rearrangement of habit.

Once you have this new form of cooking blended into

your routine, there are several cookbooks designed for specific weight loss diets, diabetic slow cooking, or even going Vegetarian.  A crock pot is one of the most fabulous appliances that you can own.  Follow the 5-day plan for putting menus in place and discover that you have more time than you did by opening a box and preparing the contents.  You will find yourself switching to healthier foods, saving on groceries, and using less energy.

The crock pot can be an essential part of your life when you realize the multiple advantages it provides in cooking.  Keep this book handy and learn why crock pot cooking is making such a popular come back.  You will discover that the crock pot has always been a valuable tool, but perhaps, a little ahead of its time, for being noticed and appreciated.

CPSIA information can be obtained
at www.ICGtesting.com
Printed in the USA
BVOW11s1410301117

501625BV00025B/1635/P